Yoga Teacher Planner

Name :

Address:

Phone:

Email:

Yoga Teacher Planner

Date

Time

Venue

Theme/Focus:

Props

Oils

Music

No. Of
Attendees:

Private class: y / n

Note

- ○
- ○
- ○
- ○
- ○
- ○
- ○
- ○

Feedback

☆ ☆ ☆ ☆ ☆

Mantra / Positive Quote:

Yoga Teacher Planner

Date

Time

Venue

Theme/Focus:

Props . . . .
. . . .
. . . .
. . . .
. . . .
. . . .
. . . .
. . . .
. . . .
. . . .

Oils   Music

No. Of
Attendees:

Private class: y / n

Note
○
○
○
○
○
○
○
○

Feedback

☆ ☆ ☆ ☆ ☆

Mantra / Positive Quote:

Yoga Teacher Planner

Date

Time

Venue

Theme/Focus:

Props

Oils

Music

No. Of
Attendees:

Private class: y / n

Note

○
○
○
○
○
○
○
○

Feedback

☆ ☆ ☆ ☆ ☆

Mantra / Positive Quote:

Yoga Teacher Planner

Date

Time

Venue

Theme/Focus:

Props

Oils

Music

No. Of
Attendees:

Private class: y / n

Note

◯
◯
◯
◯
◯
◯
◯
◯

Feedback

☆ ☆ ☆ ☆ ☆

Mantra / Positive Quote:

Yoga Teacher Planner

Date

Time

Venue

Theme/Focus:

Props

Oils

Music

No. Of
Attendees:

Private class: y / n

Note

- ◯
- ◯
- ◯
- ◯
- ◯
- ◯
- ◯
- ◯

Feedback

☆ ☆ ☆ ☆ ☆

Mantra / Positive Quote:

Yoga Teacher Planner

Date

Time

Venue

Theme/Focus:

Props

. . . .

Oils

Music

No. Of
Attendees:

Private class: y / n

Note

○
○
○
○
○
○
○
○

Feedback

☆ ☆ ☆ ☆ ☆

Mantra / Positive Quote:

Yoga Teacher Planner

Date

Time

Venue

Theme/Focus:

Props

Oils

Music

No. Of Attendees:

Private class: y / n

Note

○
○
○
○
○
○
○
○

Feedback

☆ ☆ ☆ ☆ ☆

Mantra / Positive Quote:

Yoga Teacher Planner

Date

Time

Venue

Theme/Focus:

Props . . . .

Oils

Music

No. Of
Attendees:

Private class: y / n

Note

- ○
- ○
- ○
- ○
- ○
- ○
- ○
- ○

Feedback

☆ ☆ ☆ ☆ ☆

Mantra / Positive Quote:

Yoga Teacher Planner

Date

Time

Venue

Theme/Focus:

Props

. . . .

. . . .

. . . .

. . . .

. . . .

. . . .

. . . .

. . . .

. . . .

. . . .

Oils

Music

No. Of Attendees:

Private class: y / n

Note

○ ______________________
○ ______________________
○ ______________________
○ ______________________
○ ______________________
○ ______________________
○ ______________________
○ ______________________

Feedback

☆ ☆ ☆ ☆ ☆

Mantra / Positive Quote:

Yoga Teacher Planner

Date

Time

Venue

Theme/Focus:

Props

Oils

Music

No. Of
Attendees:

Private class: y / n

Note

-
-
-
-
-
-
-
-

Feedback

☆ ☆ ☆ ☆ ☆

Mantra / Positive Quote:

Yoga Teacher Planner

Date

Time

Venue

Theme/Focus:

Props . . . .

Oils

Music

No. Of
Attendees:

Private class: y / n

Note

○
○
○
○
○
○
○
○

Feedback

☆ ☆ ☆ ☆ ☆

Mantra / Positive Quote:

Yoga Teacher Planner

Date

Time

Venue

Theme/Focus:

Props

Oils

Music

No. Of Attendees:

Private class: y / n

Note

- ◯
- ◯
- ◯
- ◯
- ◯
- ◯
- ◯
- ◯

Feedback

☆ ☆ ☆ ☆ ☆

Mantra / Positive Quote:

Yoga Teacher Planner

Date ....

Time ....

Venue ....

Theme/Focus: ....

Props

Oils

Music

No. Of
Attendees: ....

Private class: y / n

Note

○ ....
○ ....
○ ....
○ ....
○ ....
○ ....
○ ....
○ ....

Feedback

☆ ☆ ☆ ☆ ☆

Mantra / Positive Quote:

Yoga Teacher Planner

Date

Time

Venue

Theme/Focus:

Props

Oils

Music

No. Of Attendees:

Private class: y / n

Note

-
-
-
-
-
-
-
-

Feedback

☆ ☆ ☆ ☆ ☆

Mantra / Positive Quote:

Yoga Teacher Planner

Date

Time

Venue

Theme/Focus:

Props

Oils

Music

No. Of Attendees:

Private class: y / n

Note

○
○
○
○
○
○
○
○

Feedback

☆ ☆ ☆ ☆ ☆

Mantra / Positive Quote:

Yoga Teacher Planner

Date

Time

Venue

Theme/Focus:

Props

Oils

Music

No. Of Attendees:

Private class: y / n

Note

○
○
○
○
○
○
○
○

Feedback

☆ ☆ ☆ ☆ ☆

Mantra / Positive Quote:

Yoga Teacher Planner

Date

Time

Venue

Theme/Focus:

Props

Oils

Music

No. Of Attendees:

Private class: y / n

Note

- ○
- ○
- ○
- ○
- ○
- ○
- ○
- ○

Feedback

☆ ☆ ☆ ☆ ☆

Mantra / Positive Quote:

Yoga Teacher Planner

Date

Time

Venue

Theme/Focus:

Props

Oils

Music

No. Of
Attendees:

Private class: y / n

Note

○
○
○
○
○
○
○
○

Feedback

☆ ☆ ☆ ☆ ☆

Mantra / Positive Quote:

Yoga Teacher Planner

Date

Time

Venue

Theme/Focus:

Props . . . .

Oils

Music

No. Of
Attendees:

Private class: y / n

Note

- ○
- ○
- ○
- ○
- ○
- ○
- ○
- ○

Feedback

☆ ☆ ☆ ☆ ☆

Mantra / Positive Quote:

Yoga Teacher Planner

Date

Time

Venue

Theme/Focus:

Props

Oils

Music

No. Of
Attendees:

Private class: y / n

Note

○
○
○
○
○
○
○
○

Feedback

☆ ☆ ☆ ☆ ☆

Mantra / Positive Quote:

Yoga Teacher Planner

Date

Time

Venue

Theme/Focus:

Props

Oils

Music

No. Of
Attendees:

Private class: y / n

Note

- ○
- ○
- ○
- ○
- ○
- ○
- ○
- ○

Feedback

☆ ☆ ☆ ☆ ☆

Mantra / Positive Quote:

Yoga Teacher Planner

Date

Time

Venue

Theme/Focus:

Props . . . .

Oils

Music

No. Of
Attendees:

Private class: y / n

Note

- ○
- ○
- ○
- ○
- ○
- ○
- ○
- ○

Feedback

☆ ☆ ☆ ☆ ☆

Mantra / Positive Quote:

Yoga Teacher Planner

Date

Time

Venue

Theme/Focus:

Props

Oils

Music

No. Of Attendees:

Private class: y / n

Note

○
○
○
○
○
○
○
○

Feedback

☆ ☆ ☆ ☆ ☆

Mantra / Positive Quote:

Yoga Teacher Planner

Date

Time

Venue

Theme/Focus:

Props . . . .
. . . .
. . . .
. . . .
. . . .
. . . .
. . . .
. . . .
. . . .
. . . .

Oils

Music

No. Of Attendees:

Private class: y / n

Note

○

○

○

○

○

○

○

○

Feedback

☆ ☆ ☆ ☆ ☆

Mantra / Positive Quote:

Yoga Teacher Planner

Date

Time

Venue

Theme/Focus:

Props

Oils

Music

No. Of
Attendees:

Private class: y / n

Note

Feedback

☆ ☆ ☆ ☆ ☆

Mantra / Positive Quote:

Yoga Teacher Planner

Date

Time

Venue

Theme/Focus:

Props . . . .

Oils

Music

No. Of
Attendees:

Private class: y / n

Note

○
○
○
○
○
○
○
○

Feedback

☆ ☆ ☆ ☆ ☆

Mantra / Positive Quote:

Yoga Teacher Planner

Date

Time

Venue

Theme/Focus:

Props . . . .

Oils

Music

No. Of Attendees:

Private class: y / n

Note

○ ____________
○ ____________
○ ____________
○ ____________
○ ____________
○ ____________
○ ____________
○ ____________

Feedback

☆ ☆ ☆ ☆ ☆

Mantra / Positive Quote:

Yoga Teacher Planner

Date

Time

Venue

Theme/Focus:

Props

Oils

Music

No. Of
Attendees:

Private class: y / n

Note

○
○
○
○
○
○
○
○

Feedback

☆ ☆ ☆ ☆ ☆

Mantra / Positive Quote:

Yoga Teacher Planner

Date

Time

Venue

Theme/Focus:

Props

Oils

Music

No. Of
Attendees:

Private class: y / n

Note

Feedback

☆ ☆ ☆ ☆ ☆

Mantra / Positive Quote:

Yoga Teacher Planner

Date

Time

Venue

Theme/Focus:

Props . . . .

Oils

Music

No. Of
Attendees:

Private class: y / n

Note

○
○
○
○
○
○
○
○

Feedback

☆ ☆ ☆ ☆ ☆

Mantra / Positive Quote:

Yoga Teacher Planner

Date

Time

Venue

Theme/Focus:

Props

Oils

Music

No. Of Attendees:

Private class: y / n

Note

- ○
- ○
- ○
- ○
- ○
- ○
- ○
- ○

Feedback

☆ ☆ ☆ ☆ ☆

Mantra / Positive Quote:

Yoga Teacher Planner

Date

Time

Venue

Theme/Focus:

Props . . . .

Oils

Music

No. Of Attendees:

Private class: y / n

Note

- ○
- ○
- ○
- ○
- ○
- ○
- ○
- ○

Feedback

☆ ☆ ☆ ☆ ☆

Mantra / Positive Quote:

Yoga Teacher Planner

Date

Time

Venue

Theme/Focus:

Props

Oils

Music

No. Of
Attendees:

Private class: y / n

Note

-
-
-
-
-
-
-
-

Feedback

☆ ☆ ☆ ☆ ☆

Mantra / Positive Quote:

Yoga Teacher Planner

Date ....

Time ....

Venue ....

Theme/Focus: ....

....

Props . . . .
. . . .
. . . .
. . . .
. . . .
. . . .
. . . .
. . . .
. . . .

Oils

Music

No. Of
Attendees: ....

Private class: y / n

Note

○ __________________
○ __________________
○ __________________
○ __________________
○ __________________
○ __________________
○ __________________
○ __________________

Feedback

☆ ☆ ☆ ☆ ☆

Mantra / Positive Quote:

Yoga Teacher Planner

Date

Time

Venue

Theme/Focus:

Props

Oils

Music

No. Of Attendees:

Private class: y / n

Note

- ○
- ○
- ○
- ○
- ○
- ○
- ○
- ○

Feedback

☆ ☆ ☆ ☆ ☆

Mantra / Positive Quote:

Yoga Teacher Planner

Date

Time

Venue

Theme/Focus:

Props

Oils

Music

No. Of
Attendees:

Private class: y / n

Note

○
○
○
○
○
○
○
○

Feedback

☆ ☆ ☆ ☆ ☆

Mantra / Positive Quote:

Yoga Teacher Planner

Date

Time

Venue

Theme/Focus:

Props

Oils

Music

No. Of Attendees:

Private class: y / n

Note

-
-
-
-
-
-
-
-

Feedback

☆ ☆ ☆ ☆ ☆

Mantra / Positive Quote:

Yoga Teacher Planner

Date

Time

Venue

Theme/Focus:

Props

Oils

Music

No. Of Attendees:

Private class: y / n

Note

○
○
○
○
○
○
○
○

Feedback

☆ ☆ ☆ ☆ ☆

Mantra / Positive Quote:

Yoga Teacher Planner

Date

Time

Venue

Theme/Focus:

Props ·

Oils

Music

No. Of
Attendees:

Private class: y / n

Note

- ○
- ○
- ○
- ○
- ○
- ○
- ○
- ○

Feedback

☆ ☆ ☆ ☆ ☆

Mantra / Positive Quote:

Yoga Teacher Planner

Date

Time

Venue

Theme/Focus:

Props . . . .
. . . .
. . . .
. . . .
. . . .
. . . .
. . . .
. . . .
. . . .

Oils

Music

No. Of Attendees:

Private class: y / n

Note

○ _______________
○ _______________
○ _______________
○ _______________
○ _______________
○ _______________
○ _______________
○ _______________

Feedback

☆ ☆ ☆ ☆ ☆

Mantra / Positive Quote:

Yoga Teacher Planner

Date

Time

Venue

Theme/Focus:

Props

Oils

Music

No. Of
Attendees:

Private class: y / n

Note

○
○
○
○
○
○
○
○

Feedback

☆ ☆ ☆ ☆ ☆

Mantra / Positive Quote:

Yoga Teacher Planner

Date ___________________

Time ___________________

Venue __________________

Theme/Focus: ___________________
____
____

Props . . . .
. . . .
. . . .
. . . .
. . . .
. . . .
. . . .
. . . .
. . . .
. . . .

Oils

Music

No. Of
Attendees: ___________

Private class: y / n

Note

○ ___________________
○ ___________________
○ ___________________
○ ___________________
○ ___________________
○ ___________________
○ ___________________
○ ___________________

Feedback

☆ ☆ ☆ ☆ ☆

Mantra / Positive Quote:

Yoga Teacher Planner

Date

Time

Venue

Theme/Focus:

Props

Oils

Music

No. Of Attendees:

Private class: y / n

Note

○
○
○
○
○
○
○
○

Feedback

☆ ☆ ☆ ☆ ☆

Mantra / Positive Quote:

Yoga Teacher Planner

Date

Time

Venue

Theme/Focus:

Props

Oils

Music

No. Of
Attendees:

Private class: y / n

Note

○
○
○
○
○
○
○
○

Feedback

☆ ☆ ☆ ☆ ☆

Mantra / Positive Quote:

Yoga Teacher Planner

Date

Time

Venue

Theme/Focus:

Props

Oils

Music

No. Of Attendees:

Private class: y / n

Note

- ○
- ○
- ○
- ○
- ○
- ○
- ○
- ○

Feedback

☆ ☆ ☆ ☆ ☆

Mantra / Positive Quote:

Yoga Teacher Planner

Date

Time

Venue

Theme/Focus:

Props

Oils

Music

No. Of
Attendees:

Private class: y / n

Note

○
○
○
○
○
○
○
○

Feedback

☆ ☆ ☆ ☆ ☆

Mantra / Positive Quote:

Yoga Teacher Planner

Date

Time

Venue

Theme/Focus:

Props

Oils

Music

No. Of
Attendees:

Private class: y / n

Note

○
○
○
○
○
○
○
○

Feedback

☆ ☆ ☆ ☆ ☆

Mantra / Positive Quote:

Yoga Teacher Planner

Date

Time

Venue

Theme/Focus:

Props

Oils

Music

No. Of
Attendees:

Private class: y / n

Note

- ○
- ○
- ○
- ○
- ○
- ○
- ○
- ○

Feedback

☆ ☆ ☆ ☆ ☆

Mantra / Positive Quote:

Yoga Teacher Planner

Date

Time

Venue

Theme/Focus:

Props . . . .

Oils

Music

No. Of Attendees:

Private class: y / n

Note

- ○
- ○
- ○
- ○
- ○
- ○
- ○
- ○

Feedback

☆ ☆ ☆ ☆ ☆

Mantra / Positive Quote:

Yoga Teacher Planner

Date

Time

Venue

Theme/Focus:

Props

Oils

Music

No. Of
Attendees:

Private class: y / n

Note

- ○
- ○
- ○
- ○
- ○
- ○
- ○
- ○

Feedback

☆ ☆ ☆ ☆ ☆

Mantra / Positive Quote:

Yoga Teacher Planner

Date

Time

Venue

Theme/Focus:

Props

Oils

Music

No. Of
Attendees:

Private class: y / n

Note

-
-
-
-
-
-
-
-

Feedback

☆ ☆ ☆ ☆ ☆

Mantra / Positive Quote:

Yoga Teacher Planner

Date

Time

Venue

Theme/Focus:

Props . . . .

Oils

Music

No. Of Attendees:

Private class: y / n

Note

○
○
○
○
○
○
○
○

Feedback

☆ ☆ ☆ ☆ ☆

Mantra / Positive Quote:

Yoga Teacher Planner

Date

Time

Venue

Theme/Focus:

Props

Oils

Music

No. Of
Attendees:

Private class: y / n

Note

○
○
○
○
○
○
○
○

Feedback

☆ ☆ ☆ ☆ ☆

Mantra / Positive Quote:

Yoga Teacher Planner

Date

Time

Venue

Theme/Focus:

Props . . . .

Oils

Music

No. Of
Attendees:

Private class: y / n

Note

○

○

○

○

○

○

○

○

Feedback

☆ ☆ ☆ ☆ ☆

Mantra / Positive Quote:

Yoga Teacher Planner

Date

Time

Venue

Theme/Focus:

Props . . . .
. . . .
. . . .
. . . .
. . . .
. . . .
. . . .
. . . .
. . . .
. . . .

Oils

Music

No. Of Attendees:

Private class: y / n

Note

○
○
○
○
○
○
○
○

Feedback

☆ ☆ ☆ ☆ ☆

Mantra / Positive Quote:

Yoga Teacher Planner

Date

Time

Venue

Theme/Focus:

Props . . . .
. . . .
. . . .
. . . .
. . . .
. . . .
. . . .
. . . .
. . . .
. . . .
. . . .

Oils

Music

No. Of Attendees:

Private class: y / n

Note

○
○
○
○
○
○
○
○

Feedback

☆ ☆ ☆ ☆ ☆

Mantra / Positive Quote:

Yoga Teacher Planner

Date

Time

Venue

Theme/Focus:

Props

Oils

Music

No. Of Attendees:

Private class: y / n

Note

○
○
○
○
○
○
○
○

Feedback

☆ ☆ ☆ ☆ ☆

Mantra / Positive Quote:

Yoga Teacher Planner

Date

Time

Venue

Theme/Focus:

Props . . . .

Oils

Music

No. Of Attendees:

Private class: y / n

Note

- ○
- ○
- ○
- ○
- ○
- ○
- ○
- ○

Feedback

☆ ☆ ☆ ☆ ☆

Mantra / Positive Quote:

Yoga Teacher Planner

Date

Time

Venue

Theme/Focus:

Props

Oils

Music

No. Of
Attendees:

Private class: y / n

Note

- ○
- ○
- ○
- ○
- ○
- ○
- ○
- ○

Feedback

☆ ☆ ☆ ☆ ☆

Mantra / Positive Quote:

Yoga Teacher Planner

Date

Time

Venue

Theme/Focus:

Props

Oils

Music

No. Of
Attendees:

Private class: y / n

Note

○
○
○
○
○
○
○
○

Feedback

☆ ☆ ☆ ☆ ☆

Mantra / Positive Quote:

Yoga Teacher Planner

Date

Time

Venue

Theme/Focus:

Props

Oils

Music

No. Of Attendees:

Private class: y / n

Note

- ○
- ○
- ○
- ○
- ○
- ○
- ○
- ○

Feedback

☆ ☆ ☆ ☆ ☆

Mantra / Positive Quote:

Yoga Teacher Planner

Date

Time

Venue

Theme/Focus:

Props

Oils

Music

No. Of Attendees:

Private class: y / n

Note

○ ________
○ ________
○ ________
○ ________
○ ________
○ ________
○ ________
○ ________

Feedback

☆ ☆ ☆ ☆ ☆

Mantra / Positive Quote:

Yoga Teacher Planner

Date

Time

Venue

Theme/Focus:

Props

Oils

Music

No. Of
Attendees:

Private class: y / n

Note

○
○
○
○
○
○
○
○

Feedback

☆ ☆ ☆ ☆ ☆

Mantra / Positive Quote:

Yoga Teacher Planner

Date

Time

Venue

Theme/Focus:

Props

Oils

Music

No. Of
Attendees:

Private class: y / n

Note

- ○
- ○
- ○
- ○
- ○
- ○
- ○
- ○

Feedback

☆ ☆ ☆ ☆ ☆

Mantra / Positive Quote:

Yoga Teacher Planner

Date

Time

Venue

Theme/Focus:

Props . . . .

Oils

Music

No. Of Attendees:

Private class: y / n

Note

○
○
○
○
○
○
○
○

Feedback

☆ ☆ ☆ ☆ ☆

Mantra / Positive Quote:

Yoga Teacher Planner

Date

Time

Venue

Theme/Focus:

Props . . . .

Oils

Music

No. Of
Attendees:

Private class: y / n

Note

- ○
- ○
- ○
- ○
- ○
- ○
- ○
- ○

Feedback

☆ ☆ ☆ ☆ ☆

Mantra / Positive Quote:

Yoga Teacher Planner

Date ....

Time ....

Venue ....

Theme/Focus: ....

....

....

Props . . . .

. . . .

. . . .

. . . .

. . . .

. . . .

. . . .

. . . .

Oils   **Music**

No. Of Attendees: ....

Private class: y / n

Note

○ ——————————————
○ ——————————————
○ ——————————————
○ ——————————————
○ ——————————————
○ ——————————————
○ ——————————————
○ ——————————————

Feedback

☆ ☆ ☆ ☆ ☆

Mantra / Positive Quote:

Yoga Teacher Planner

Date

Time

Venue

Theme/Focus:

Props

Oils

Music

No. Of
Attendees:

Private class: y / n

Note

Feedback

☆ ☆ ☆ ☆ ☆

Mantra / Positive Quote:

Yoga Teacher Planner

Date

Time

Venue

Theme/Focus:

Props

Oils

Music

No. Of Attendees:

Private class: y / n

Note

- ○
- ○
- ○
- ○
- ○
- ○
- ○
- ○

Feedback

☆ ☆ ☆ ☆ ☆

Mantra / Positive Quote:

Yoga Teacher Planner

Date

Time

Venue

Theme/Focus:

Props

Oils

Music

No. Of
Attendees:

Private class: y / n

Note

Feedback

☆ ☆ ☆ ☆ ☆

Mantra / Positive Quote:

Yoga Teacher Planner

Date

Time

Venue

Theme/Focus:

Props

Oils

Music

No. Of
Attendees:

Private class: y / n

Note

○
○
○
○
○
○
○
○

Feedback

☆ ☆ ☆ ☆ ☆

Mantra / Positive Quote:

Yoga Teacher Planner

Date

Time

Venue

Theme/Focus:

Props

Oils

Music

No. Of
Attendees:

Private class: y / n

Note

○
○
○
○
○
○
○
○

Feedback

☆ ☆ ☆ ☆ ☆

Mantra / Positive Quote:

Yoga Teacher Planner

Date

Time

Venue

Theme/Focus:

Props

Oils

Music

No. Of
Attendees:

Private class: y / n

Note

- ◯
- ◯
- ◯
- ◯
- ◯
- ◯
- ◯
- ◯

Feedback

☆ ☆ ☆ ☆ ☆

Mantra / Positive Quote:

Yoga Teacher Planner

Date

Time

Venue

Theme/Focus:

Props

Oils

Music

No. Of
Attendees:

Private class: y / n

Note

○
○
○
○
○
○
○
○

Feedback

☆ ☆ ☆ ☆ ☆

Mantra / Positive Quote:

Yoga Teacher Planner

Date

Time

Venue

Theme/Focus:

Props

Oils

Music

No. Of Attendees:

Private class: y / n

Note

Feedback

☆ ☆ ☆ ☆ ☆

Mantra / Positive Quote:

Yoga Teacher Planner

Date

Time

Venue

Theme/Focus:

Props

Oils

Music

No. Of
Attendees:

Private class: y / n

Note

○
○
○
○
○
○
○
○

Feedback

☆ ☆ ☆ ☆ ☆

Mantra / Positive Quote:

Yoga Teacher Planner

Date

Time

Venue

Theme/Focus:

Props

Oils

Music

No. Of
Attendees:

Private class: y / n

Note

- ◯
- ◯
- ◯
- ◯
- ◯
- ◯
- ◯
- ◯

Feedback

☆ ☆ ☆ ☆ ☆

Mantra / Positive Quote:

Yoga Teacher Planner

Date

Time

Venue

Theme/Focus:

Props

Oils

Music

No. Of Attendees:

Private class: y / n

Note

○

○

○

○

○

○

○

○

Feedback

☆ ☆ ☆ ☆ ☆

Mantra / Positive Quote:

Yoga Teacher Planner

Date

Time

Venue

Theme/Focus:

Props

Oils

Music

No. Of Attendees:

Private class: y / n

Note

○
○
○
○
○
○
○
○

Feedback

☆ ☆ ☆ ☆ ☆

Mantra / Positive Quote:

Yoga Teacher Planner

Date

Time

Venue

Theme/Focus:

Props

Oils

Music

No. Of Attendees:

Private class: y / n

Note

○
○
○
○
○
○
○
○

Feedback

☆ ☆ ☆ ☆ ☆

Mantra / Positive Quote:

Yoga Teacher Planner

Date ....

Time ....

Venue ....

Theme/Focus: ....

Props ·

Oils   **Music**

No. Of Attendees:

Private class: y / n

Note

○ ___________________________
○ ___________________________
○ ___________________________
○ ___________________________
○ ___________________________
○ ___________________________
○ ___________________________
○ ___________________________

Feedback

☆ ☆ ☆ ☆ ☆

Mantra / Positive Quote:

Yoga Teacher Planner

Date

Time

Venue

Theme/Focus:

Props . . . .

. . . .

. . . .

. . . .

. . . .

. . . .

. . . .

. . . .

. . . .

. . . .

Oils

Music

No. Of Attendees:

Private class: y / n

Note

- ○
- ○
- ○
- ○
- ○
- ○
- ○
- ○

Feedback

☆ ☆ ☆ ☆ ☆

Mantra / Positive Quote:

Yoga Teacher Planner

Date

Time

Venue

Theme/Focus:

Props . . . .

Oils

Music

No. Of Attendees:

Private class: y / n

Note

○ ————————
○ ————————
○ ————————
○ ————————
○ ————————
○ ————————
○ ————————
○ ————————

Feedback

☆ ☆ ☆ ☆ ☆

Mantra / Positive Quote:

Yoga Teacher Planner

Date

Time

Venue

Theme/Focus:

Props

Oils

Music

No. Of
Attendees:

Private class: y / n

Note

○ ____________
○ ____________
○ ____________
○ ____________
○ ____________
○ ____________
○ ____________
○ ____________

Feedback

☆ ☆ ☆ ☆ ☆

Mantra / Positive Quote:

Yoga Teacher Planner

Date

Time

Venue

Theme/Focus:

Props

Oils   **Music**

No. Of
Attendees:

Private class: y / n

Note

○
○
○
○
○
○
○
○

Feedback

☆ ☆ ☆ ☆ ☆

Mantra / Positive Quote:

Yoga Teacher Planner

Date

Time

Venue

Theme/Focus:

Props . . . .

Oils

Music

No. Of Attendees:

Private class: y / n

Note

○
○
○
○
○
○
○
○

Feedback

☆ ☆ ☆ ☆ ☆

Mantra / Positive Quote:

Yoga Teacher Planner

Date

Time

Venue

Theme/Focus:

Props

Oils

Music

No. Of
Attendees:

Private class: y / n

Note

- ◯
- ◯
- ◯
- ◯
- ◯
- ◯
- ◯
- ◯

Feedback

☆ ☆ ☆ ☆ ☆

Mantra / Positive Quote:

Yoga Teacher Planner

Date

Time

Venue

Theme/Focus:

Props

Oils

Music

No. Of
Attendees:

Private class: y / n

Note

○
○
○
○
○
○
○
○

Feedback

☆ ☆ ☆ ☆ ☆

Mantra / Positive Quote:

Yoga Teacher Planner

Date

Time

Venue

Theme/Focus:

Props

Oils

Music

No. Of
Attendees:

Private class: y / n

Note

○
○
○
○
○
○
○
○

Feedback

☆ ☆ ☆ ☆ ☆

Mantra / Positive Quote:

Yoga Teacher Planner

Date

Time

Venue

Theme/Focus:

Props

Oils

Music

No. Of Attendees:

Private class: y / n

Note

- ○
- ○
- ○
- ○
- ○
- ○
- ○
- ○

Feedback

☆ ☆ ☆ ☆ ☆

Mantra / Positive Quote:

Yoga Teacher Planner

Date

Time

Venue

Theme/Focus:

Props

Oils

Music

No. Of
Attendees:

Private class: y / n

Note

○
○
○
○
○
○
○
○

Feedback

☆ ☆ ☆ ☆ ☆

Mantra / Positive Quote:

Yoga Teacher Planner

Date

Time

Venue

Theme/Focus:

Props . . . .
. . . .
. . . .
. . . .
. . . .
. . . .
. . . .
. . . .
. . . .
. . . .

Oils

Music

No. Of Attendees:

Private class: y / n

Note

○ _______________
○ _______________
○ _______________
○ _______________
○ _______________
○ _______________
○ _______________
○ _______________

Feedback

☆ ☆ ☆ ☆ ☆

Mantra / Positive Quote:

Yoga Teacher Planner

Date

Time

Venue

Theme/Focus:

Props . . . .

Oils

Music

No. Of
Attendees:

Private class: y / n

Note

- ○
- ○
- ○
- ○
- ○
- ○
- ○
- ○

Feedback

☆ ☆ ☆ ☆ ☆

Mantra / Positive Quote:

Yoga Teacher Planner

Date

Time

Venue

Theme/Focus:

Props . . . .
. . . .
. . . .
. . . .
. . . .
. . . .
. . . .
. . . .
. . . .

Oils

Music

No. Of Attendees:

Private class: y / n

Note

○
○
○
○
○
○
○
○

Feedback

☆ ☆ ☆ ☆ ☆

Mantra / Positive Quote:

Yoga Teacher Planner

Date

Time

Venue

Theme/Focus:

Props

Oils

Music

No. Of Attendees:

Private class: y / n

Note

○
○
○
○
○
○
○
○

Feedback

☆ ☆ ☆ ☆ ☆

Mantra / Positive Quote:

Yoga Teacher Planner

Date _______________________

Time _______________________

Venue ______________________

Theme/Focus: _____________

____

____

Props . . . .
. . . .
. . . .
. . . .
. . . .
. . . .
. . . .
. . . .
. . . .
. . . .

Oils   **Music**

____

____

____

____

____

No. Of Attendees: _______________

Private class: y / n

Note

○ _______________________
○ _______________________
○ _______________________
○ _______________________
○ _______________________
○ _______________________
○ _______________________
○ _______________________

Feedback

____

____

____

____

☆ ☆ ☆ ☆ ☆

Mantra / Positive Quote:

____

____

____

____

Yoga Teacher Planner

Date

Time

Venue

Theme/Focus:

Props

Oils

Music

No. Of
Attendees:

Private class: y / n

Note

○
○
○
○
○
○
○
○

Feedback

☆ ☆ ☆ ☆ ☆

Mantra / Positive Quote:

Yoga Teacher Planner

Date

Time

Venue

Theme/Focus:

Props ·

Oils

Music

No. Of Attendees:

Private class: y / n

Note

- ○
- ○
- ○
- ○
- ○
- ○
- ○
- ○

Feedback

☆ ☆ ☆ ☆ ☆

Mantra / Positive Quote:

Yoga Teacher Planner

Date

Time

Venue

Theme/Focus:

Props . . . .

Oils

Music

Yoga Teacher Planner

Date

Time

Venue

Theme/Focus:

Props . . . .
. . . .
. . . .
. . . .
. . . .
. . . .
. . . .
. . . .
. . . .

Oils　　　　　　　　　　　**Music**

No. Of Attendees:

Private class:　y / n

Note

○ _______________
○ _______________
○ _______________
○ _______________
○ _______________
○ _______________
○ _______________
○ _______________

Feedback

☆ ☆ ☆ ☆ ☆

Mantra / Positive Quote:

Yoga Teacher Planner

Date

Time

Venue

Theme/Focus:

Props

Oils

Music

No. Of
Attendees:

Private class: y / n

Note

- ○
- ○
- ○
- ○
- ○
- ○
- ○
- ○

Feedback

☆ ☆ ☆ ☆ ☆

Mantra / Positive Quote:

Yoga Teacher Planner

Date

Time

Venue

Theme/Focus:

Props

Oils

Music

No. Of
Attendees:

Private class: y / n

Note

○
○
○
○
○
○
○
○

Feedback

☆ ☆ ☆ ☆ ☆

Mantra / Positive Quote:

Yoga Teacher Planner

Date

Time

Venue

Theme/Focus:

Props . . . .

Oils

Music

No. Of
Attendees:

Private class: y / n

Note

○
○
○
○
○
○
○
○

Feedback

☆ ☆ ☆ ☆ ☆

Mantra / Positive Quote:

Yoga Teacher Planner

Date

Time

Venue

Theme/Focus:

Props

Oils

Music

No. Of Attendees:

Private class: y / n

Note

○
○
○
○
○
○
○
○

Feedback

☆ ☆ ☆ ☆ ☆

Mantra / Positive Quote:

Yoga Teacher Planner

Date

Time

Venue

Theme/Focus:

Props

Oils

Music

No. Of Attendees:

Private class: y / n

Note

○
○
○
○
○
○
○
○

Feedback

☆ ☆ ☆ ☆ ☆

Mantra / Positive Quote:

Yoga Teacher Planner

Date

Time

Venue

Theme/Focus:

Props

Oils

Music

No. Of
Attendees:

Private class: y / n

Note

○
○
○
○
○
○
○
○

Feedback

☆ ☆ ☆ ☆ ☆

Mantra / Positive Quote:

Yoga Teacher Planner

Date

Time

Venue

Theme/Focus:

Props

Oils

Music

No. Of
Attendees:

Private class: y / n

Note

○
○
○
○
○
○
○
○

Feedback

☆ ☆ ☆ ☆ ☆

Mantra / Positive Quote:

Yoga Teacher Planner

Date

Time

Venue

Theme/Focus:

Props

Oils

Music

No. Of Attendees:

Private class: y / n

Note

○

○

○

○

○

○

○

○

Feedback

☆ ☆ ☆ ☆ ☆

Mantra / Positive Quote:

Yoga Teacher Planner

Date

Time

Venue

Theme/Focus:

Props . . . .

Oils

Music

No. Of
Attendees:

Private class: y / n

Note

○
○
○
○
○
○
○
○

Feedback

☆ ☆ ☆ ☆ ☆

Mantra / Positive Quote:

Yoga Teacher Planner

Date

Time

Venue

Theme/Focus:

Props

Oils

Music

No. Of
Attendees:

Private class: y / n

Note

- ○
- ○
- ○
- ○
- ○
- ○
- ○
- ○

Feedback

☆ ☆ ☆ ☆ ☆

Mantra / Positive Quote:

Yoga Teacher Planner

Date

Time

Venue

Theme/Focus:

Props . . . .

Oils

Music

No. Of
Attendees:

Private class: y / n

Note

- ○ ____________
- ○ ____________
- ○ ____________
- ○ ____________
- ○ ____________
- ○ ____________
- ○ ____________
- ○ ____________

Feedback

☆ ☆ ☆ ☆ ☆

Mantra / Positive Quote:

Yoga Teacher Planner

Date

Time

Venue

Theme/Focus:

Props

Oils

Music

No. Of Attendees:

Private class: y / n

Note

○
○
○
○
○
○
○
○

Feedback

☆ ☆ ☆ ☆ ☆

Mantra / Positive Quote:

Yoga Teacher Planner

Date

Time

Venue

Theme/Focus:

Props

Oils

Music

No. Of Attendees:

Private class: y / n

Note

- ○
- ○
- ○
- ○
- ○
- ○
- ○
- ○

Feedback

☆ ☆ ☆ ☆ ☆

Mantra / Positive Quote:

Yoga Teacher Planner

Date

Time

Venue

Theme/Focus:

Props . . . .

Oils

Music

No. Of
Attendees:

Private class: y / n

Note

○
○
○
○
○
○
○
○

Feedback

☆ ☆ ☆ ☆ ☆

Mantra / Positive Quote:

Yoga Teacher Planner

Date

Time

Venue

Theme/Focus:

Props

Oils

Music

No. Of
Attendees:

Private class: y / n

Note

-
-
-
-
-
-
-
-

Feedback

☆ ☆ ☆ ☆ ☆

Mantra / Positive Quote:

Yoga Teacher Planner

Date

Time

Venue

Theme/Focus:

Props . . . .
. . . .
. . . .
. . . .
. . . .
. . . .
. . . .
. . . .
. . . .
. . . .
. . . .

Oils

Music

No. Of Attendees:

Private class: y / n

Note

○
○
○
○
○
○
○
○

Feedback

☆ ☆ ☆ ☆ ☆

Mantra / Positive Quote:

Yoga Teacher Planner

Date

Time

Venue

Theme/Focus:

Props

Oils

Music

No. Of Attendees:

Private class: y / n

Note

- ○
- ○
- ○
- ○
- ○
- ○
- ○
- ○

Feedback

☆ ☆ ☆ ☆ ☆

Mantra / Positive Quote:

Yoga Teacher Planner

Date

Time

Venue

Theme/Focus:

Props

Oils

Music

No. Of Attendees:

Private class: y / n

Note

-
-
-
-
-
-
-
-

Feedback

☆ ☆ ☆ ☆ ☆

Mantra / Positive Quote:

Yoga Teacher Planner

Date

Time

Venue

Theme/Focus:

Props

Oils

Music

No. Of
Attendees:

Private class: y / n

Note

○
○
○
○
○
○
○
○

Feedback

☆ ☆ ☆ ☆ ☆

Mantra / Positive Quote:

Yoga Teacher Planner

Date

Time

Venue

Theme/Focus:

Props . . . .
. . . .
. . . .
. . . .
. . . .
. . . .
. . . .
. . . .
. . . .
. . . .
. . . .
. . . .

Oils   **Music**

No. Of Attendees:

Private class: y / n

Note

○
○
○
○
○
○
○
○

Feedback

☆ ☆ ☆ ☆ ☆

Mantra / Positive Quote:

Yoga Teacher Planner

Date

Time

Venue

Theme/Focus:

Props

Oils

Music

No. Of Attendees:

Private class: y / n

Note
- ○
- ○
- ○
- ○
- ○
- ○
- ○
- ○

Feedback

☆ ☆ ☆ ☆ ☆

Mantra / Positive Quote:

Yoga Teacher Planner

Date

Time

Venue

Theme/Focus:

Props

Oils

Music

No. Of
Attendees:

Private class: y / n

Note

○
○
○
○
○
○
○
○

Feedback

☆ ☆ ☆ ☆ ☆

Mantra / Positive Quote:

Yoga Teacher Planner

Date

Time

Venue

Theme/Focus:

Props

Oils

Music

No. Of Attendees:

Private class: y / n

Note

-
-
-
-
-
-
-
-

Feedback

☆ ☆ ☆ ☆ ☆

Mantra / Positive Quote:

Yoga Teacher Planner

Date

Time

Venue

Theme/Focus:

Props . . . .

Oils

Music

No. Of
Attendees:

Private class: y / n

Note

○
○
○
○
○
○
○
○

Feedback

☆ ☆ ☆ ☆ ☆

Mantra / Positive Quote:

Yoga Teacher Planner

Date

Time

Venue

Theme/Focus:

Props

Oils

Music

No. Of Attendees:

Private class: y / n

Note

- ○
- ○
- ○
- ○
- ○
- ○
- ○
- ○

Feedback

☆ ☆ ☆ ☆ ☆

Mantra / Positive Quote:

Yoga Teacher Planner

Date

Time

Venue

Theme/Focus:

Props . . . .
. . . .
. . . .
. . . .
. . . .
. . . .
. . . .
. . . .
. . . .

Oils

Music

No. Of Attendees:

Private class: y / n

Note

○
○
○
○
○
○
○
○
○

Feedback

☆ ☆ ☆ ☆ ☆

Mantra / Positive Quote:

Yoga Teacher Planner

Date

Time

Venue

Theme/Focus:

Props . . . .
. . . .
. . . .
. . . .
. . . .
. . . .
. . . .
. . . .
. . . .
. . . .

Oils   **Music**

No. Of Attendees:

Private class: y / n

Note

○ ——————————
○ ——————————
○ ——————————
○ ——————————
○ ——————————
○ ——————————
○ ——————————
○ ——————————

Feedback

☆ ☆ ☆ ☆ ☆

Mantra / Positive Quote:

Yoga Teacher Planner

Date

Time

Venue

Theme/Focus:

Props . . . .

Oils

Music

No. Of Attendees:

Private class: y / n

Note

○
○
○
○
○
○
○
○
○

Feedback

☆ ☆ ☆ ☆ ☆

Mantra / Positive Quote:

Yoga Teacher Planner

Date

Time

Venue

Theme/Focus:

Props

Oils

Music

No. Of Attendees:

Private class: y / n

Note

- ○
- ○
- ○
- ○
- ○
- ○
- ○
- ○

Feedback

☆ ☆ ☆ ☆ ☆

Mantra / Positive Quote:

Yoga Teacher Planner

Date

Time

Venue

Theme/Focus:

Props

Oils

Music

No. Of
Attendees:

Private class: y / n

Note

Feedback

☆ ☆ ☆ ☆ ☆

Mantra / Positive Quote: